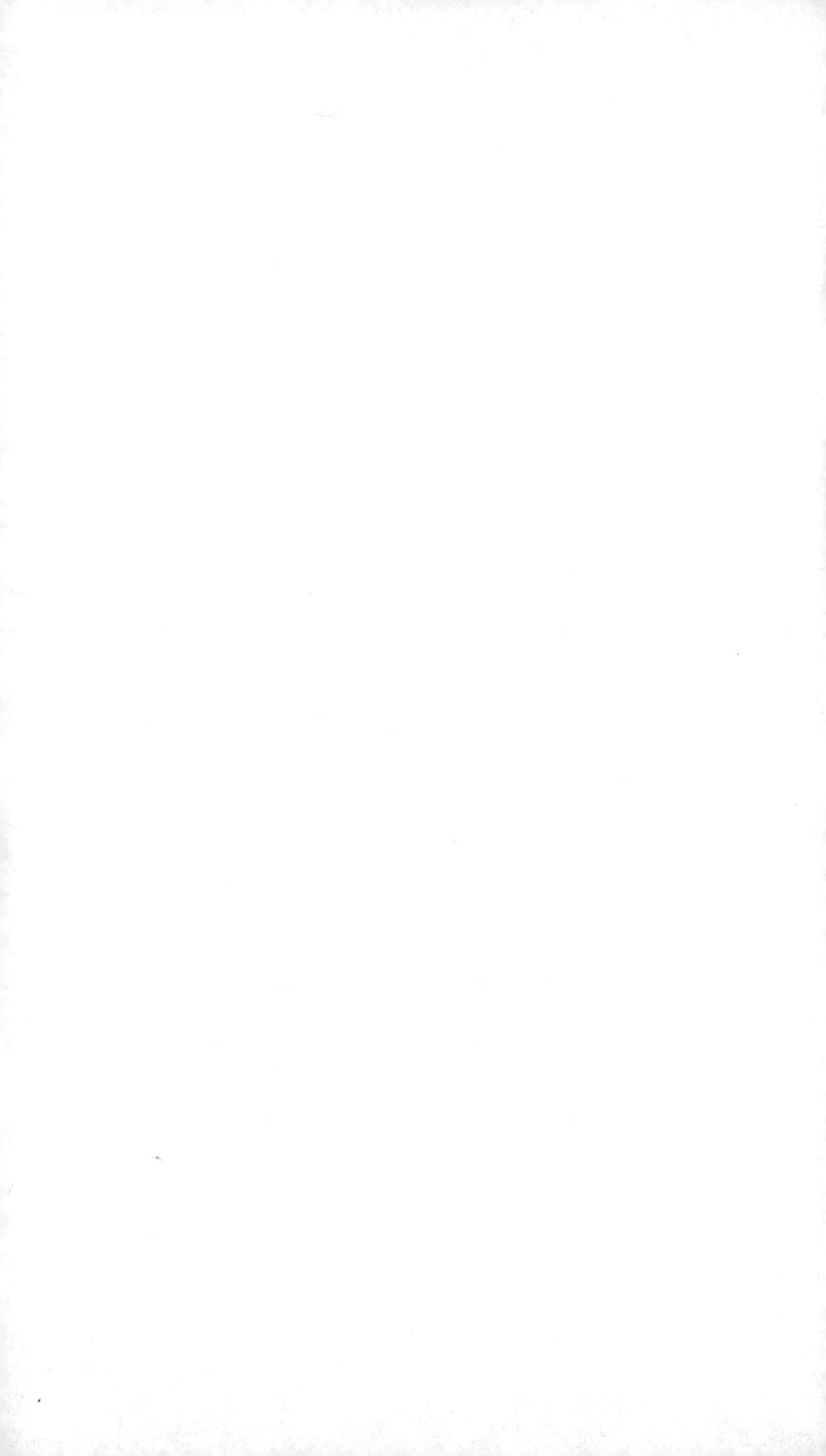

THE ULTIMATE WATCH YOUR WEIGHT COOKBOOK FOR BALANCED LIVING 2024

WW Beginners Top Recipes: An Experienced Guide To a Balanced Diet, Slim and Fit Body.

By

Nicole J. Deleon

Copyright

© Copyright 2024 by Nicole J. Deleon. All rights reserved.

No part of The Ultimate Watch Your Weight Cookbook for Balanced Living 2024 may be reproduced, distributed, or transmitted in any form or by any means, including photocopying, recording, or other electronic or mechanical techniques, without the publisher's prior written consent, with the exception of brief quotations used in critical reviews and other nonprofit uses that are allowed by copyright law.

Disclaimer:

The information provided on The Ultimate Watch Your Weight Cookbook for Balanced Living 2024 is for general informational purposes only. Although we make every effort to provide accurate and up-to-date information, we do not make any express or implied representations or warranties about the correctness, dependability, suitability, or availability of The Ultimate Watch Your Weight Cookbook for Balanced Living 2024 or the information, products, services, or related graphics contained on The Ultimate Watch Your Weight Cookbook for Balanced Living 2024 for any purpose. Any reliance on this material is sorely at your own risk. We are not responsible for any loss of data or profits, resulting from using The Ultimate Watch Your Weight Cookbook for Balanced Living 2024.

About the author

Hey, lovely readers! I'm Nicole J. Deleon, your culinary companion and a bit of a food enthusiast on a journey to discover the perfect harmony between deliciousness and healthy living.

Now, let me spill the beans – I'm all about weight watching and healthy eating, not because it's a fad, but because it's a journey. I believe in creating dishes that whisper tales of balance, where the joy of eating meets the wisdom of nourishing your body.

You know, I've spent countless hours tinkering in the kitchen, testing recipes, and yes, having a few delightful kitchen mishaps along the way. But that's the beauty of it – cooking is an adventure, and each meal is a chance to explore, create, and indulge in the pleasure of good food.

So, as you flip through these pages, think of me as your culinary friend who's cheering you on to savor the goodness, make healthier choices, and revel in the simple joy of eating well. Let's embark on this delightful journey together, where every bite is a step towards a healthier, happier you!

Table of contents

INTRODUCTION

Welcome to the culinary adventure to a better, more energetic self! We set out on a delightful journey that blends the pleasure of eating with the knowledge of making wise decisions in this Watch Your Weight Cookbook. This collection of dishes is intended to make every meal an opportunity for nourishment and satisfaction, regardless of your experience level with the Watch your Weight program. The idea of SmartPoints, a tool that enables you to choose your food with awareness, is the foundation of our journey. You'll find that eating healthy doesn't have to mean compromising flavor or fun as we go through a range of breakfasts, lunches, dinners, snacks, and sweet delights. Finding the ideal balance that suits you is more important. This cookbook is a guide to creating a long-term and meaningful relationship with food, not just a collection of recipes. We'll discuss meal preparation, offer advice on how to set your kitchen for success, and different food recipes for the Watch your Weight way of life. Now let's get started, enjoy every bite, and go in the direction of a happy, healthier you. Cheers to a world of delicious opportunities that satisfy the body and the spirit. Let's toast to mindful eating and a journey full of flavour and health!

Overview of the Watch Your Weight Program:

The Watch Your Weight program is all about making healthy living simple, enjoyable, and sustainable. It's more than just a diet; it's a means to change how you think about food, activity, and well-being in a way that integrates smoothly into your daily routine.

Picture this: You're enjoying your favorite meals, still indulging in that occasional slice of pizza or piece of chocolate, and yet, you're steadily moving towards your health goals. That's the beauty of the Watch Your Weight program. It's designed to help you lose weight without feeling like you're constantly fighting against cravings or depriving yourself of the foods you love.

This program focuses on making tiny, practicable changes to achieve long-term success. Instead of making sudden changes that can be difficult to maintain, you'll gradually learn to make better choices. These choices over time can result in long-term weight loss and a better lifestyle.

One of the most fascinating aspects of the Watch Your Weight program is how everything is tailored to your specific needs. We all have different bodies, tastes, and routines, so why should we all eat the same way? This program takes into account your age, weight, height, activity level, and personal preferences to build a plan that feels customized just for you. This way, you're more likely to stick with it because it doesn't feel like a one-size-fits-all approach.

Flexibility is an important aspect of this program. You don't have to give up your social life or avoid eating out. You'll learn how to make smarter choices at home, while dining out, or even on vacation. It is about finding balance and enjoying life while working towards your health goals.

Support is another key aspect of the Watch Your Weight program. You're not in this alone. Whether you prefer attending local workshops, connecting with an online community, or using the comprehensive app, there's a network of people ready to cheer you on and share their tips and experiences. This sense of community can make a huge difference, providing motivation and accountability.

But it's not all about food. Watch Your Weight program takes a comprehensive approach to health. It promotes consistent physical activity, mindful eating, and healthy habits that improve your mental and emotional well-being. It's about creating a balanced, healthy lifestyle that you can maintain for the long haul, not just for a few weeks or months.

This program offers a lot of educational resources. You'll have access to healthy recipes, meal plans, and recommendations for various eating situations. Whether you're packing lunch for work, planning a family dinner, or ordering at a restaurant, you'll have the expertise and knowledge to make smarter choices.

The Watch Your Weight program is all about fitting healthy habits into your life in a way that feels natural and sustainable. It's about enjoying food, staying active, and feeling good about yourself. With this program, you're setting off on a path to a healthier, happier you—one small, positive step at a time. Welcome to a new way of living that's delicious, balanced, and totally achievable.

Understanding SmartPoints and How They Work:

Alright, let's talk SmartPoints – your sidekick in the delicious journey of wellness. Imagine them as your personalized nutrition compass, guiding you through the sea of food choices. Here's the lowdown on how these little wonders work:

Every Food Earns a score: Each food item gets its very own SmartPoints value. It's not just about calories – SmartPoints consider the protein, carbs, fats, and sugars, giving you a holistic view of what you're munching on.

Tailored to You: Forget generic plans. Your SmartPoints budget is as unique as you are. Your age, weight, height, and activity level shape this budget, making it a custom-fit guide for your daily eats.

Budget Your Bites: Think of SmartPoints as your daily spending limit for food. Fancy a burger? Sure, but it'll take a chunk out of your SmartPoints budget. Load up on veggies? They're the budget-friendly stars of your plate.

Embrace the Variety: No food is banished from the kingdom of SmartPoints. From a slice of pizza to a colorful salad, if it fits your SmartPoints budget, it's a winner. It's about finding balance and keeping things interesting.

Rollover Perks: Missed the mark on a particular day? Fear not! You've got Weekly SmartPoints in your pocket – a safety net for those occasional indulgences or spontaneous cravings.

Track, Don't Slack: The real magic happens when you track your SmartPoints. Whether through the app or a trusty journal, it's not about restriction; it's about awareness. Tracking helps you make savvy choices and stay on the path to your goals.

In a nutshell, SmartPoints are your GPS to healthier eating. They guide you in crafting meals that not only tantalize your taste buds but also align with your wellness ambitions. So, dive into the SmartPoints universe and let the journey to a tastier, balanced lifestyle commence!

CHAPTER 1: GETTING STARTED

Setting Up Your Kitchen for Success:

Creating a kitchen that supports your wellness goals is a game-changer. Here's a roadmap to set up your culinary space for success:

Organize Your Pantry:

Arrange your pantry with essentials like whole grains, legumes, canned tomatoes, and healthy cooking oils. A well-organized pantry makes meal preparation smoother.

Stock Up on Smart Snacks:

Keep smart snack options on hand, such as nuts, seeds, and fresh fruits. Having these readily available can help curb unhealthy cravings.

Invest in Quality Cookware:

Quality pots, pans, and utensils make cooking more enjoyable and efficient. Non-stick cookware can reduce the need for excessive oils

Fill Your Fridge with Fresh Produce:

Keep a variety of fresh fruits and vegetables in your fridge. Colorful and nutrient-rich produce is the foundation of a healthy diet.

Herbs and Spices Galore:

Build a collection of herbs and spices to add flavor without extra calories. Ditch the salt and experiment with herbs like rosemary, thyme, and cumin.

Smart Storage Solutions:

Invest in storage containers to keep leftovers fresh and portion sizes in check. Meal planning is made simpler and food waste is decreased as a result.

Choose Whole Grains:

Choose whole grains such as whole wheat pasta, quinoa, and brown rice. When compared to processed grains, these offer more fiber and minerals.

Protein Power:

Stock up on lean protein sources such as chicken breast, tofu, beans, and fish. Having these options readily available ensures balanced and satisfying meals.

Healthy Cooking Oils:

Choose heart-healthy oils like olive oil or avocado oil for cooking. These fats add flavor and are beneficial for your overall health.

Mindful Eating Tools:

Invest in smaller plates and bowls to encourage portion control. Being mindful of your serving sizes can contribute to weight management.

Smart Appliances:

Consider appliances like a blender for smoothies, a steamer for veggies, or an air fryer for healthier cooking methods.

Hydration Station:

Keep a water dispenser or pitcher in plain sight. It's important to stay hydrated for general health and to manage appetite.

Meal Prep containers:

Meals can be prepared ahead of time and kept in portion-controlled containers. This makes it easy to grab a healthy option when time is limited.

Guide to Nutritional Information:

Have a reference manual on SmartPoints values close at hand. This aids in the decision-making process while planning and cooking meals.

By arranging your kitchen in this way, you can provide a supportive environment for your Watch Your Weight journey, which will help you maintain your goals and prepare a wide range of delicious healthful meals. Setting up your kitchen with these elements creates a supportive environment for your Watch Your Weight journey, making it easier to stay on track and enjoy a variety of delicious, wholesome meals.

Tips for Meal Planning and Prep:

Create a Weekly Menu:

Plan your meals for the week ahead. Include a mix of protein, vegetables, whole grains, and healthy fats. This helps you stay organized and reduces the temptation to make last-minute unhealthy choices.

Consider SmartPoints:

Factor in SmartPoints values when planning your meals. This ensures you're mindful of your daily and weekly budgets, helping you make balanced choices.

Batch Cooking:

Prepare larger quantities of certain recipes and portion them for multiple meals. This saves time during the week and ensures you have healthy options readily available.

Mix and Match Ingredients:

Opt for versatile ingredients that can be used in several meals throughout the week. For example, roasted veggies can be added to salads, wraps, or grain bowls.

Prep Fresh Fruits and Vegetables:

Wash, chop, and portion fruits and veggies at the beginning of the week. Having them ready to go makes it easier to incorporate them into meals and snacks.

Utilize Freezer-Friendly Meals:

Prepare freezer-friendly meals in advance. Soups, stews, and casseroles often freeze well and can be reheated for quick and convenient dinners.

Plan for Leftovers:

Embrace leftovers as planned meals. Cook extra portions, and enjoy them the next day for lunch or dinner. It reduces cooking time and minimizes food waste.

Smart Snack Prep:

Have healthy snacks prepped and portioned. This avoids reaching for less nutritious options when hunger strikes between meals.

Build a Spice Collection:

Invest in a variety of spices to add flavor without extra calories. Experimenting with different spices can make your meals more interesting.

Schedule Weekly Prep Time:

Dedicate a specific time each week to meal planning and prep. Consistency is key, and having a routine makes it a sustainable habit.

Try Theme Nights:

Assign specific themes to different nights of the week, like Meatless Mondays or Taco Tuesdays. This adds variety and simplifies decision-making.

Prep Breakfasts in Advance:

Overnight oats, yogurt parfaits, or pre-made smoothie packs can streamline your morning routine and ensure a nutritious start to the day.

Invest in Quality Storage Containers:

Use a variety of containers for meal storage, including portion-sized containers for snacks. This allows you to easily grab meals on the go.

Stay Flexible:

Be open to adjustments in your plan. Life happens, and flexibility is essential. Have backup options for busier days.

 Meal planning and preparation are effective techniques for remaining on track with your Weight Watchers goals. By using these suggestions, you can save time, make better choices, and position yourself for success in accomplishing your wellness objectives.

CHAPTER 2:

BREAKFAST RECIPES

1) Mini Egg Muffins with Spinach and Feta:

- Prep time: 10 minutes
- Cook time: 20 minutes
- Total time: 30 minutes
- Servings: 12
- Smart points: 2

INGREDIENTS

- 2 Tbsp. olive oil
- ½ a red onion, finely chopped
- 2-3 big handfuls of spinach, chopped
- 12 large eggs
- 1 cup of crumbled feta
- Salt and pepper to taste

- ½ tsp. dried oregano

INSTRUCTION

1. Preheat the oven to 350°F. Brush a 12-cup non-stick muffin tin with olive oil—you can also use cupcake liners if you prefer or a silicon muffin tin.

2. Fill a pan with one tablespoon of olive oil and set it over medium heat. . When the onions are transparent, add them to the skillet and move them to a bowl.

3. In the same skillet, cook the chopped spinach for about 2-3 minutes until it wilts. Remove any remaining water from the spinach, place it in the same bowl as your onions, and let it cool.

4. Crack all 12 eggs into a large mixing dish of your choice and beat them.. Add half of the crumbled feta and salt, pepper, and oregano. Add the spinach and onions after that.

5. Spoon the egg mixture equally into each muffin cup, then sprinkle the remaining feta cheese over the top of the frittatas. . Bake for about 20 minutes until the tops are firm.

6. Remove carefully from the oven and allow the mini frittatas to cool off before removing from the muffin tin.

7. Store in an airtight container in your fridge for four to five days.

NUTRITIONAL FACTS

- Calories: 128 kcal
- Carbohydrates: 2g
- Protein: 8g
- Fat: 10g

2) Scrambled Eggs with Tomatoes and Spinach :

- Prep time: 5 minutes
- Cook time : 5 minutes
- Total time: 10 minutes
- Servings: 2
- Smart points: 3

INGREDIENTS

- 1 tbsp olive oil, plus 1 tsp
- 3 tomatoes, halved
- 4 large eggs
- 4 tbsp natural bio yogurt
- ⅓ small pack basil, chopped
- 175g of baby spinach, well-dried (wash if necessary).

INSTRUCTION

1. In a big, nonstick frying pan, heat up 1 tsp oil. Add the tomatoes and cook over medium heat, cut-side down.

2. While they are cooking, beat the eggs in a jug with the yogurt, 2 tbsp water, plenty of black pepper and the basil.

3. Transfer the tomatoes to serving plates. Add the spinach to the pan and wilt, stirring a few times while you cook the eggs.

4. Heat the rest of the oil in a non-stick pan over a medium heat, pour in the egg mixture and stir every now and then until scrambled and just set.

5. After spooning the spinach onto the plates, place the scrambled eggs on top..

NUTRITIONAL FACTS

- Calories: 297 kcal

- Carbohydrate: 10g

- Protein: 20g

- Fat: 20g

3) Breakfast Burrito with Black Beans and Veggie Scramble:

- Prep time: 10 minute
- Cook time: 15 minutes
- Total time: 25 minutes
- Servings: 2
- Smart points: 4

INGREDIENTS

- 2 Tortillas
- 4 eggs, scrambled
- Pinch each salt and pepper
- 4 tsp (20 mL) butter
- 3/4 cup (175 mL) black beans
- 1/2 cup (125 mL) Monterey Jack cheese
- 1/2 avocado, halved, pitted, peeled and sliced
- 1/4 cup (60 mL) tomato salsa
- 2 tbsp (30 mL) finely chopped fresh cilantro

INSTRUCTIONS

1. Add 1 tbsp (15 mL) water, salt, and pepper to beat eggs.

2. Melt butter in a nonstick skillet set over medium heat; pour in egg mixture.

3. Cook for about 5 minutes, stirring often, or until soft curds form and the eggs are set.

4. Place a little border at either end of each tortilla and spoon scrambled eggs down the center of each one.

5. Top with beans, cheese, avocado, salsa and cilantro.

6. Tightly roll the tortilla by folding in the edges and covering the contents with the bottom.

NUTRITIONAL FACTS

- Calories: 300 kcal
- Carbohydrates: 30g
- Protein: 10g
- Fat: 10g

4) Blueberry Oatmeal with Chia Seeds and Nuts:

- Prep time: 5 minutes
- Cook time: 15 minutes
- Total time: 20 minutes
- Serving: 4
- Smart points: 4

INGREDIENTS

- 2 cups rolled oats gluten-free
- 3 tablespoons chia seeds
- 2 teaspoons vanilla extract
- pinch of sea salt
- 1 cup blueberries
- 2 tablespoons honey or 100% maple syrup to make it vegan
- 4 cups almond milk unsweeteend
- 1 tablespoon lemon

INSTRUCTIONS

1. Put all the ingredients in a medium-sized saucepan and cook it on medium-high until it boils.

2. After reducing heat to medium, cook oatmeal for approximately ten minutes, stirring often, until most of the liquid has been absorbed and the oatmeal has thickened..

3. Top with walnuts and fresh blueberries.

NUTRITIONAL FACTS

- Calories: 248 kcal
- Carbohydrates:43g
- Protein:7g
- Fat: 6g

5) Baked Sweet Potato with Greek Yogurt and Cinnamon:

- Prep time: 15 minutes
- Cook time: 10 minutes
- Total time: 25 minutes
- Servings: 4
- Smart points: 3

INGREDIENTS

- 4 small to medium Sweet Potatoes baked
- 5.3 oz Greek Yogurt Plain or Vanilla
- 2 teaspoons Honey
- ½ teaspoon Cinnamon
- ¼ teaspoon Vanilla
- ½ cup chopped Pecans toasted

INSTRUCTIONS

1. In a small bowl, combine yogurt, honey, cinnamon and vanilla.

2. Split open sweet potatoes and fill each one with a little of the yogurt mixture.

3. Mix into potato to combine well.

4. Divide pecans between potatoes and serve hot.

NUTRITIONAL FACTS

- Calories: 240 kcal
- Carbohydrates: 32g
- Protein: 7g
- Fat: 10g

6) Greek Yogurt Parfait with Fruit and Granola:

- Prep time: 11 minutes
- Total time: 11 minutes
- Servings: 4
- Smart points: 3

INGREDIENTS

- 2 cups Greek yogurt, your favorite flavor!
- 2 cups granola
- 1 cup fresh blueberries, rinsed
- 1 cup fresh strawberries, rinsed, hulled, and cut into fourths
- cup fresh pineapple, diced
- Four to eight-ounce glasses or mason jars

INSTRUCTIONS

1. Pour about a quarter of a cup of the yogurt into your glass.

2. On top of the yogurt, add approximately ¼ cup of the granola.

3. Sprinkle about ¼ cup of the blueberries over the granola.

4. Continue from steps 1-3 until all the fruits are in the glass or container.

NUTRITIONAL FACTS

- Calories: 300 kcal
- Carbohydrates: 40g
- Protein: 20g
- Fat: 10g

CHAPTER 3: LUNCH RECIPES

1) One-Pan Lemon Garlic Roasted Chicken with Asparagus:

- Prep time: 10 minutes
- Cook time: 40 minutes
- Total time: 50 minutes
- Servings: 6
- Smart points: 2

INGREDIENTS

- Six skin-or bone-in chicken thighs
- Pinch of salt to season
- Cracked black pepper
- Two tsp dried thyme, or any other preferred herb

- 1 tablespoon olive oil
- 2 tablespoons unsalted butter
- Six smashed garlic cloves, or one and a half teaspoons of minced garlic
- Juice of 1 lemon (about 1/3 cup fresh squeezed lemon juice)

INSTRUCTIONS

1. Preheat your oven to 200°C | 400° F. Add dried thyme, salt, and pepper to chicken thighs for seasoning.
2. Over medium-high heat, preheat a large (34 cm or 13–14 inch) cast iron skillet (or heavy-based oven-proof pan).
3. Add the oil to the heated skillet (or pan). Sear the thighs for about 4–5 minutes, with the skin side down, or until the skin is crisp and golden.
4. Sear the chicken for a further five minutes after flipping it over..

5. Melt the butter in the pan. Sauté the garlic for about 30 seconds, or until fragrant.

6. Add the lemon juice, garnish with the fresh leaves from two sprigs of thyme. Add two more sprigs to the chicken's surround.

7. Place the skillet (or pan) in the oven and cook it for twenty to thirty minutes, or until it's cooked through. In the final 12 minutes of cooking, add the asparagus spears to the pan.

8. Add lemon slices and the remaining sprig of thyme's leaves as garnish. Serve immediately.

NUTRITIONAL FACTS

- Calories: 321 kcal
- Carbohydrates: 3g
- Protein: 35g
- Fat: 17g

2) Turkey Taco Lettuce Wraps:

- Prep time: 5 minutes
- Cook time: 10 minutes
- Total time: 15 minutes
- Servings: 6
- Smart points: 4

INGREDIENTS

- 1 1/4 lb 99% fat-free lean ground turkey
- 1 1/2 tsp chili powder
- 1 tsp cumin
- 1 tsp dried oregano
- 1/4 tsp salt
- 1 (15 oz) can diced tomatoes, drained
- 1 (4.5 oz) can chopped green chiles
- 1 cup fresh or frozen corn
- 1 (15 oz) can black beans, drained and rinsed
- 1/2 cup (or more) chunky salsa
- 2 Tbsp chopped cilantro

- Juice of half a lime
- 12 butter lettuce leaves
- Toppings (optional): shredded cheese, avocado, sour cream

INSTRUCTIONS

1. Cook the ground turkey in a big pan over medium heat until it starts to crumble and get browned.

2. Cook the turkey until it is well cooked and browned, adding more cumin, oregano, and chili powder as needed.

3. Add the corn, black beans, tomatoes, green chilies, salsa, and cilantro and stir.

4. After cooking for a further five minutes or so, add the lime juice and heat through.

5. To each lettuce cup, pour about 1/4 cup of the turkey mixtureAdd your favorite toppings on top, then dig in !

NUTRITIONAL FACTS

- Calories: 194 kcal
- Carbohydrates: 24.4g
- Protein: 23.3g
- Fat: 1.4g

3) Lentil Soup with Whole-Wheat Bread:

- Prep time: 10 minutes
- Cook time: 40 minutes
- Total time: 50 minutes
- Servings: 4
- Smart points: 4

INGREDIENTS

- 2 cups lentils
- 1 tablespoon extra virgin olive oil
- 2 carrots, peeled and chopped
- 2 celery ribs, thinly sliced
- ½ yellow onion, diced
- 8 ounces cremini mushrooms, thinly sliced
- 2 garlic cloves, minced
- 1 ½ cups coarsely chopped packaged laciento kale

- 1 teaspoon herbs de provence or Italian seasoning
- 5 cups vegetable broth/chicken broth (+ about 2 cups of water added during cooking)
- ¼ cup white wine
- ½ cup unsweetened coconut milk
- 1 teaspoon lemon juice
- To taste, add coarse salt and ground black pepper.

FOR THE CROUTONS

- One pound of artisanal whole grain bread (I used French bread)
- ¼ cup olive oil
- ¼ teaspoon salt
- ¼ teaspoon ground black pepper

INSTRUCTIONS

1. Make the croutons: Preheat oven to 375°F. Slice the bread into ½ inch slices. Tear slices into bite sized pieces.

2. Spread the bread cubes with salt, pepper, and olive oil in a big bowl. Toss to combine.

3.   Place the croutons in a single layer on a baking sheet after pouring them over. Bake for 15 to 20 minutes, or until browned, rotating the croutons halfway through to ensure equal toasting. . Set aside to cool.

4. While the croutons are baking, heat olive oil in a large pot over medium high heat. Add onion, celery, mushrooms and carrots. Cook for 5-7 minutes until veggies have softened and mushrooms have started to release juices.

5. Add garlic and cook 1 minute, until fragrant. Pour white wine into the pan, scraping any browned bits off the bottom of the pan.

6. Add lentils, herbs, and broth. Bring to a boil, cover, and reduce to a simmer. Cook for 35-45 minutes until lentils are tender, pouring in water as needed to make sure lentils are always just covered with liquid.

7. Remove from heat and stir in kale, coconut milk, and lemon juice, stirring to combine. Add salt and black pepper to taste. Top with cooled croutons to serve.

NUTRITIONAL FACTS

- Calories: 400 kcal
- Carbohydrates: 65g
- Protein:20g
- Fat: 7g

4) Air Fryer Salmon with Lemon Dill Sauce:

- Prep time: 2 minutes
- Cook time: 8 minutes
- Total time: 10 minutes
- Servings: 4
- Smart points: 5

INGREDIENTS

- 4X120g/4 oz salmon filets
- salt and pepper
- 1 lemon, juice and zest
- cooking spray
- 125g/1/2 cup mayonnaise can use low fat
- 1 tsp Dijon mustard
- 1 tbsp chopped dill

INSTRUCTIONS

1. Preheat the air fryer to 400F/200C. While the air fryer is heating up, rub the salmon all over with the zest of half a lemon and season with salt and pepper.

2. After the air fryer has been preheated, place the salmon into the basket and give it a frying spray. (If you want to use oil rather than spray, drizzle 1 tsp of olive oil over the salmon and season with salt, pepper, and lemon zest.) Prepare food for 8 minutes.

3. While the salmon is cooking, in a small bowl, mix the mayonnaise with the zest and juice of ½ lemon, mustard and chopped dill to make the sauce.

NUTRITIONAL FACTS

- Calories: 253 kcal
- Carbohydrates: 5g
- Protein: 24g
- Fat: 15g

5) Chicken Caesar Salad with Light Dressing:

- Prep time: 5 minutes
- Cook time: 25 minutes
- Total time: 30 minutes
- Servings: 4
- Smart points: 4

INGREDIENTS

- Four cups of cubed, crusty, day-old bread (ideally whole wheat)
- 2 tablespoons extra-virgin olive oil
- 1/2 cup nonfat plain Greek yogurt
- 1 cup shredded parmesan cheese (about 2 ounces)
- 1 small clove garlic
- 2 anchovy filets
- Juice of 1 lemon
- 1 teaspoon dijon mustard

- 1 pound skinless, boneless chicken breasts
- Kosher salt
- 2 romaine lettuce hearts, chopped
- Freshly ground pepper

INSTRUCTIONS

1. Prepare the croutons: Set the oven's temperature to 350°F. Toss the bread cubes in a large bowl with 1 tablespoon olive oil.

2. Spread on a baking sheet and bake until crisp, tossing halfway through, about 20 minutes.

3. Meanwhile, make the dressing: Puree the yogurt, 2 tablespoons parmesan, the garlic, anchovies, lemon juice, mustard and 2 tablespoons water in a mini food processor or a blender.

4. Pound the chicken between 2 pieces of plastic wrap with a heavy skillet until 1/2 inch thick.

5.   Brush a rimmed baking sheet with the remaining 1 tablespoon olive oil; add the chicken and season with salt.

6.   Brush evenly with 1 tablespoon of the dressing and sprinkle with 2 tablespoons of parmesan. Broil, undisturbed, until golden and cooked through, about 5 minutes.

7.   Transfer to a cutting board. In a large bowl, combine the lettuce, croutons, remaining dressing, and 3/4 cup of parmesan cheese.

8.   Thinly slice the chicken. Divide the salad among bowls, top with the chicken and season with pepper.

NUTRITIONAL FACTS

- Calories: 368 kcal
- Carbohydrates: 21g
- Protein: 37g
- Fat: 15g

6) Shrimp Scampi with Zucchini Noodles:

- Prep time: 10 minutes
- Cook time: 5 minutes
- Total time: 15 minutes
- Servings: 5
- Smart points: 5

INGREDIENTS

- 2 tablespoons butter
- 3 garlic cloves minced
- ¼ teaspoon crushed red pepper
- 2 pounds shrimp shelled and deveined
- Salt and pepper
- 1 teaspoon paprika
- ½ cup vegetable broth
- ¼ cup red wine vinegar
- Juice of a lemon
- 3 zucchinis spiralized

- Shaved Parmesan cheese for serving
- Fresh parsley for serving

INSTRUCTIONS

1. Heat the butter in a big pan, then add the crushed red pepper and garlic until aromatic, for one minute.

2. When the shrimp become pink, which should take two to four minutes depending on their size, add them to the pan and season with salt, pepper, and paprika. Using a slotted spoon, remove the shrimp.

3. The remaining sauce in the pan can be thickened somewhat by adding the vegetable broth, red wine vinegar, and lemon juice while scraping down the sides of the pan.

4. After turning off the heat, mix the shrimp and spiralized zucchini to reheat them just a bit. If preferred, garnish with freshly chopped parsley and Parmesan cheese.

NUTRITIONAL FACTS

- Calories: 251 kcal

- Carbohydrates: 5g

- Protein: 39g

- Fat: 7g

CHAPTER 4: DINNER RECIPES

1) Creamy One-Pot Tomato Basil Pasta with Chicken:

- Prep time: 10 minutes
- Cook time: 20 minutes
- Total time: 30 minutes
- Sevings: 4
- Smart points: 5

INGREDIENTS

- 2 Tbsp. extra-virgin olive oil
- 1 cup diced yellow onion
- 1 pint cherry tomatoes, halved
- 8 oz. dry penne pasta
- 1 cup marinara sauce
- 2 cups water

- ½ tsp. garlic powder
- ½ tsp. dried oregano
- ½ tsp. Each kosher salt and freshly ground black pepper
- two to three hearty handfuls of crisp baby spinach
- ⅓ cup heavy cream
- ½ cup shredded mozzarella cheese
- ¼ cup chopped fresh basil leaves
- Grated Parmesan cheese for garnish (optional)

INSTRUCTIONS

1. Heat 2 Tbsp.Over medium heat, add oil to a big skillet that fits with a cover.

2. Add onion and tomatoes; cook 7 to 8 minutes, until the onion is soft and tomatoes are broken down and jammy.

3. Pasta, marinara sauce, water, oregano, garlic powder, salt, and pepper should all be added.

4. Turn the heat up to medium-high and let the mixture simmer for ten to twelve minutes, or until the pasta is al dente, simmer, covered, and stir periodically.

5. Take off the cover and mix in the cheese, spinach, and heavy cream. Stir constantly for approximately two minutes, or until spinach wilts and cheese melts. If using, garnish with Parmesan and fresh basil.

NUTRITIONAL FACTS

- Calories: 447 kcal
- Carbohydrates: 54g
- Protein: 14g
- Fat: 22g

2) Turkey Meatloaf Muffins with Sweet Potato Mash:

- Prep time: 10 minutes
- Cook time: 20 minutes
- Total time,: 30 minutes
- Servings: 2
- Smart points: 4

INGREDIENTS

- 1 1/2 lb. ground beef
- 2 tsp. cooking oil (olive, coconut, or avocado oil) or ghee
- 1 small onion, minced
- 3 garlic cloves, peeled and minced
- 1/2 cup Whole30-compliant barbecue sauce
- 1 tsp. dried thyme
- 1/2 tsp. salt
- 1/2 tsp. black pepper

TOPPING:

- 2 medium sweet potatoes, peeled and cubed

- 1 Tbsp. coconut oil or ghee (you may use butter if Whole30 is not necessary for you)

- 1/4 tsp. salt

INSTRUCTIONS

1. Preheat the oven to 350°F.

2. Transfer ground beef to a medium-sized bowl and keep aside.

3. Heat the oil in a small skillet over medium heat. Add onions and cook until they begin to soften, stirring now and again.

4. Once fragrant, cook the garlic for 30 seconds.

5. Add onion-garlic mixture to ground beef. Stir in dried thyme, sea salt, pepper, and barbecue sauce. You may use your hands or a spoon to mix the ingredients.

6. Evenly distribute the meat mixture among the muffin pan's 12 wells.

7. Bake for 20 minutes, or until the meat is no longer pink in the middle, in a preheated oven.

8. Steam sweet potatoes for 10 to 12 minutes, or until they are cooked, while the meatloaves are baking. Sweet potatoes should be drained, then pureed with butter or coconut oil in a food processor, or well mashed with a fork.

9. Spread the topping over the meatloaves using a spoon, or use a plastic zip-top bag filled with topping, cut the corner with scissors, and pipe the topping over the meatloaves. Or use a spoon to top.

10. Drizzle with additional barbecue sauce, if desired.

NUTRITIONAL FACTS

- Calories: 300 kcal
- Carbohydrates: 22g
- Protein: 25g
- Fat: 12g

3) Grilled Lemon Herb Chicken with Greek Yogurt Ranch:

- Prep time: 35 minutes
- Cook time: 25 minutes
- Total time: 1hour
- Servings: 4
- Smart points: 4

INGREDIENTS

- 1 tablespoon lemon zest
- 2 tbsp fresh lemon juice
- 2 tbsp extra virgin olive oil
- 2 tbsp nonfat greek yogurt
- 3 garlic cloves minced about 1 tablespoon
- 2 tablespoons of fresh herbs chopped finely.

  I prefer a 50/50 blend of parsley and basil.
- .5 tsp salt
- .25 tsp ground black pepper

- 1.25 lbs 1 ¼ lb of skinless, boneless chicken breast

INSTRUCTIONS

1. In a medium bowl, whisk the lemon zest, lemon juice, olive oil, yogurt, garlic, parsley, salt, and pepper.

2. Fill a plastic gallon bag with the marinade, add the chicken, squeeze out as much air as you can, and close the bag. To ensure that the chicken marinates evenly, turn the bag a few times to coat the chicken with marinade.

3. Refrigerate for at least 30 minutes or up to a day, turning the bag halfway through.

4. Close the lid and preheat your gas grill using all of the burners on high. After about fifteen minutes, when the grill reaches a high temperature, turn down the two burners nearest to the front while leaving the back burner on high.

5.   Take the chicken out of the bag and place it over the low-heat burners on the grates. Cover and cook for 6 to 9 minutes, or until the underside of the chicken starts to show some light grill marks.

6. After flipping the chicken, cover it, and cook for a further 6 to 9 minutes, or until the chicken is firm to the touch.

7. Now move the chicken to the area of the grill over high flames and cook it uncovered until each side has a solid grill mark, five to six minutes flipping halfway.

8. The chicken should be completely firm to the touch and register 160 degrees F on an instant-read thermometer.

9.   Transfer the chicken to a platter, cover with foil, and let it lie for five minutes before serving.

NUTRITIONAL FACTS

- Calories: 205 kcal

- Carbohydrates: 2g

- Protein: 33g

- Fat: 7g

4) Honey Garlic Salmon with Roasted Brussels Sprouts:

- Prep time: 5 minutes
- Cook time: 30 minutes
- Total time: 35 minutes
- Servings: 4
- Smart points : 5

INGREDIENTS

- Four chopped, crushed, or grated garlic cloves
- 1/4 cup low-sodium soy sauce
- 1/3 cup honey
- freshly cracked black pepper
- 1 (2 pound) salmon filet, about 1 1/2 inches thick
- 1 pound brussels sprouts, cut in half or even quartered
- lemon wedges for spritzing

- fresh herbs, like basil, oregano, chives for topping

INSTRUCTIONS

1. Preheat the oven to 425 degrees F. Line a sheet pan with parchment paper or foil. To ensure that your Brussels sprouts roast rapidly, cut them into little pieces. I prefer to chop them into quarters after removing the stems.
2. Combine the honey, soy sauce, and garlic in a small bowl. Place the salmon filet in the center of the sheet
3. Toss the sprouts with half of the honey garlic combination after placing them in the bowl .
4. Spread the brussels around the salmon. Brush the remaining honey garlic mixture over the salmon. If you have any leftovers, that's OK; you can use it to brush on after the salmon is

finished ! I like to add some freshly cracked pepper on top too.

5. For 15 minutes, roast the salmon and Brussels sprouts, or until the fish flakes easily with a fork and the sprouts start to caramelize.

6. Remove and slice the salmon into pieces. Serve immediately with a sprinkling of herbs, a spritz of lemon and extra sauce!

NUTRITIONAL FACTS

- Calories: 450 kcal
- Carbohydrates: 30g
- Protein: 30g
- Fat: 20g

5) Coconut Curry Shrimp with Zucchini Noodles:

- Prep time: 10 minutes
- Cook time: 15 minutes
- Total time: 25 minutes
- Servings: 1
- Smart points: 4

INGREDIENTS

- 1 lb. Shrimp - peeled and deveined
- 2 Cups Zucchini Noodles - homemade or store-bought
- 3 Tbsp Sesame Oil - you can use any light oil
- For Curry:
- 3 Tbsp Thai Red Curry Paste
- 1 Can Coconut Milk
- 1 Tsp Chili Flakes
- 2 Tsp Sesame Seeds
- 1 Tsp Salt

- 1/2 Tsp Sugar - sweetener of choice

INSTRUCTIONS

1. Prep: In a bowl, add shrimp and 1 tbsp red curry paste. Mix everything and keep aside.

2. Heat a skillet and add 2 tbsp oil

3. Add red curry marinated shrimp and saute over medium flames for 3-4 minutes (until shrimps are cooked).

4. Transfer the shrimp to a plate and keep aside.

5. Heat 1 tbsp oil in the same pan.

6. Add chili flakes and saute over medium heat.

7. Add the red curry paste and cook for one minute.

8. Add the sugar, salt, and coconut milk now, and sauté everything until the red curry paste is dissolved in the coconut milk.

9. For three to four minutes, sauté this over medium-low heat.

10. Now, add cooked shrimp and zoodles.

11. Saute and let cook for 3 minutes.

12. Turn off the heat, sprinkle sesame seeds and serve hot.

NUTRITIONAL FACTS

- Calories: 486 kcal

- Carbohydrates: 11g

- Protein: 29g

- Fat: 38g

6) One Pan Moroccan Chicken and Couscous:

- Prep time: 15 minutes
- Cook time: 20 minutes
- Total time: 35 minutes
- Servings: 4
- Smart points: 5

INGREDIENTS

- One pound of skinless, boneless chicken breasts, chopped into 3/4-inch chunks
- 3 Tbsp olive oil, divided
- 1 tsp ground cumin, divided
- 1/2 tsp ground coriander, divided
- 1/2 tsp ground cinnamon, divided
- Salt and freshly ground black pepper
- 1 large red bell pepper, cored and chopped (1 1/2 cups)
- 3/4 cup chopped red onion

- 1 1/2 cups matchstick carrots
- 1 Tbsp minced garlic (3 cloves)
- 1/4 tsp turmeric
- 1 1/2 cups low-sodium chicken broth
- 1/3 cup chopped dried apricots or golden raisins
- 1 cup dry Moroccan couscous
- 2 Tbsp fresh lemon juice
- 1/2 cup Fisher Sliced Almonds
- 2 Tbsp chopped fresh cilantro
- 2 Tbsp chopped fresh mint

INSTRUCTIONS

1. In a 12-inch nonstick saute pan or deep skillet, heat up 1 tablespoon of olive oil over medium-high heat.

2. Add chicken to the pan and season with salt and pepper, 1/2 tsp cumin, 1/4 tsp coriander and 1/4 cinnamon. Cook for about 7 minutes, flipping regularly, or until cooked through.

3. To keep warm, transfer the chicken to a sheet of foil and wrap.

4. Heat remaining 2 Tbsp oil in skillet. Add in bell pepper and onion and saute 5 minutes.

5. Saute the carrots for one minute after adding the garlic, turmeric, 1/4 tsp coriander, 1/2 tsp cumin, and 1/4 tsp cinnamon.

6. After adding the apricots and chicken broth, season to taste with salt and pepper, and bring to a boil (the mixture should gently boil in the middle as well as simmer on the outside).

7. Stir in couscous then remove from heat and let rest 5 - 6 minutes until tender.

8. Stir in lemon juice, almonds, cilantro, mint, and chicken with any collected liquids (you can also add in little more broth if desired).Serve warm.

NUTRITIONAL FACTS

- Calories: 560 kcal

- Carbohydrates: 56g

- Protein: 32g

- Fat: 21g

CHAPTER 5: VEGETARIAN

1) Sweet Potato and Chickpea Curry:

- Prep time: 10 minutes

- Cook time: 30 minutes

- Total time: 40 minutes

- Servings: 4

- SmartPoints: 5

INGREDIENTS

- 1 tablespoon olive oil

- 1 onion, chopped

- 2 cloves garlic, minced

- 1 inch ginger, grated

- 1 tablespoon curry powder

- 1 teaspoon ground cumin

- 1/2 teaspoon turmeric

- 1/4 teaspoon chili flakes (optional)

- 400g (14oz) canned diced tomatoes
- 400ml (14oz) coconut milk (full-fat or light)
- 400g (14oz) canned chickpeas, drained and rinsed
- 2 medium sweet potatoes, peeled and cubed
- Salt and pepper to taste
- Cilantro or parsley, chopped (optional, for garnish)

INSTRUCTIONS

1. In a big saucepan or Dutch oven, warm up the olive oil over medium heat. Add the onion and simmer for approximately 5 minutes, or until softened.

2. Add garlic and ginger, cook for 1 minute more until fragrant.

3. Stir in curry powder, cumin, turmeric, and chili flakes (if using). Cook for 1 minute until the spices are fragrant.

4. Pour in diced tomatoes and coconut milk. Bring to a simmer, then stir in chickpeas and sweet potatoes.

5. Cover and simmer for 20-25 minutes, or until sweet potatoes are tender. Season with salt and pepper to taste.

6. Garnish with chopped cilantro or parsley (optional) and serve with rice, naan bread, or quinoa.

NUTRITIONAL FACTS

- Calories: 400 kcal
- Carbohydrates: 54g
- Protein: 15g
- Fat: 14g

2) Cauliflower Fried Rice:

- Prep Time: 20 minutes
- Cook Time:15 minutes
- Servings: 6
- SmartPoints: 4

INGREDIENTS

- 4 cups cauliflower
- Eggs (2 eggs and above)
- 1 tablespoon vegetable oil
- Vegetables : onions, carrots, peas, corn, bell peppers, mushrooms, and broccoli). Aim for about 2 cups total.
- Soy sauce (2 teaspoons at first and adjust as needed).
- Seasonings: ginger, garlic, sesame oil, and sriracha Start with 1/2 teaspoon each and adjust as needed.

- Green onions, cashews, peanuts, or pineapple chunks (optional)

INSTRUCTIONS

1. Prep the cauliflower: If using a head, grate it on the largest side of your grater or pulse it in a food processor to resemble rice grains. Set aside.

2. Scramble the eggs: Heat oil in a wok or large skillet over medium heat. The eggs should be scrambled and placed in a bowl.

3. Stir-fry the vegetables: Add your chosen vegetables to the wok and stir-fry until slightly softened and crisp-tender, about 3-5 minutes

4. Add the cauliflower: Push the vegetables to the side and add the cauliflower rice. Cook for 2-3 minutes, stirring occasionally, until slightly softened but still with a bite.

5. Combine and season: Add the scrambled eggs back to the pan and stir-fry together with the cauliflower and vegetables. Pour in the soy sauce and seasonings, stirring to combine. Adjust the taste as needed.

6. Serve and enjoy! Garnish with chopped green onions and your optional additions if using. Serve with protein like grilled chicken or shrimp for a complete meal.

NUTRITIONAL FACTS

- Calories: 200 kcal
- Fat: 10g
- Carbohydrates: 20g
- Protein: 10g

3) Black Bean and Corn Salad:

- Prep Time: 10 minutes
- Total time: 10 minutes
- Servings: 4
- SmartPoints: 3

INGREDIENTS

- 1 15-ounce can black beans, rinsed and drained
- 1 15-ounce can corn kernels, drained
- 1/2 red onion, finely chopped
- 1 red bell pepper, finely chopped
- 1/2 cup cherry tomatoes, halved
- 1/4 cup fresh cilantro, chopped
- 1/4 cup olive oil
- 2 tablespoons fresh lime juice
- 1/2 teaspoon chili powder
- 1/4 teaspoon cumin
- Salt and pepper to taste

INSTRUCTIONS

1. Prep: Rinse and drain the black beans and corn. Finely chop the red onion, bell pepper, and cherry tomatoes. Chop the fresh cilantro.

2. Combine: In a large bowl, combine the black beans, corn, red onion, bell pepper, cherry tomatoes, and cilantro.

3. Dressing: In a small bowl, whisk together the olive oil, lime juice, chili powder, cumin, salt, and pepper.

4. Toss and adjust: Pour the dressing over the salad ingredients and toss to coat evenly. Adjust the seasonings to taste.

5. Serve: Serve the salad immediately or chill it for at least 30 minutes for enhanced flavor.

NUTRITIONAL FACTS

- Calories: 200 kcal

- Fat: 8g

- Carbohydrates: 28g

- Protein: 8g

4) Roasted Vegetable Quinoa Bowl:

- Prep time: 20 minutes
- Cook time: 25 minutes
- Total time: 45 minutes
- Servings: 2
- Smart points: 5

INGREDIENTS

- For the Quinoa
- 1 ½ cups uncooked quinoa
- ½ teaspoon salt
- 2 ½ cups water
- For the Vegetables
- 1 red onion chopped
- 1 red pepper chopped
- 1 large sweet potato chopped into cubes
- 1 large yellow squash end trimmed, chopped into pieces measuring ½ inch
- 1 green pepper chopped

- 3 tablespoons olive oil
- 1 teaspoon salt
- ½ teaspoon black pepper
- ½ teaspoon garlic powder
- ½ teaspoon oregano
- chopped parsley for servin
- Tahini sauce for serving

INSTRUCTIONS

1. Cook the Quinoa. Place the quinoa in a small saucepan with water and salt.

2. Over medium-high heat, bring the mixture to a boil.. Reduce heat to a simmer and cook for fifteen minutes while covered.

3. Remove the pot from the heat. Without lifting the cover, let the quinoa lie in the pot for around five minutes so that it may absorb all of the liquid and steam. Lift the lid and mix the quinoa with a fork to separate it.

4. Roast the Vegetables. Preheat the oven to 425°F. Arrange the veggies on an 18 × 13-inch baking sheet that has a rim. Add a drizzle of olive oil and season with oregano, salt, pepper, and garlic powder.

5. Toss the veggies with your hands and spread them out into a uniform layer. Roast until fork tender 30 minutes. For an additional five minutes, broil the veggies after flipping them over.

6. Divide the quinoa among four bowls. Place the roasted veggies on top, then garnish with finely chopped fresh parsley. Top with tahini sauce and serve right away.

NUTRITIONAL FACTS

- Calories: 413 kcal
- Carbohydrates: 60g
- Protein: 11g
- Fat: 15g

5) Turkey Chili:

- Prep time: 10 minutes
- Cook time: 45 minutes
- Total time: 55 minutes
- Servings: 6
- Smart points: 5

INGREDIENTS

- 2 teaspoons olive oil
- 1 yellow onion, chopped
- 3 garlic cloves, minced
- 1 medium red bell pepper, chopped
- One pound of extremely lean ground chicken or turkey (99%)
- Four teaspoons of chile powder* (I used the mild McCormick variety). Avoid using hot chili powder and begin with two teaspoons if you're using a different brand.
- 2 teaspoons ground cumin

- 1 teaspoon dried oregano
- 1/4 teaspoon cayenne pepper
- 1/2 teaspoon salt, plus more to taste
- 1 (28-ounce) can of chopped or crushed tomatoes
- 1 1/4 cups chicken broth
- 2 (15 oz) cans dark red kidney beans, rinsed and drained
- 1(15-ounce)can of washed and drained sweet corn
- Topping options include cheese, avocado, sour cream, tortilla chips, cilantro.

INSTRUCTIONS

1. Fill a big saucepan with oil and heat it to a medium-high temperature. Stirring constantly, sauté the onion, garlic, and red pepper for five to seven minutes.

2. Break up the meat and add the ground turkey. Cook until the flesh is no longer pink. Add

the salt, cayenne pepper, oregano, cumin, chili powder, and mix for about 20 seconds.

3. Corn, kidney beans, tomatoes, and chicken broth should then be added. Once the chili thickens and the flavors mix together, bring it to a boil, then lower the heat and simmer it for 30 to 45 minutes. If required, taste and adjust salt and spices.

4. Garnish with anything you'd like. Makes 6 servings, about 1 1/2 cups each.

NUTRITIONAL FACTS

- Calories: 336 kcal
- Carbohydrates: 46.7g
- Protein: 31.8g
- Fat: 3.7g

CHAPTER 6: APPETIZER

1) Skinny Caprese Bites:

- Prep time: 10 minutes
- Total time: 10 minutes
- Servings: 6
- Smart points:1

INGREDIENTS

- 1/2 Small Cantaloupe
- 1.5 Oz. Prosciutto
- 8 Oz. Fresh Mozzarella
- 2 Tbsp. Light or Skinny Pesto
- 12 Fresh Basil Leaves

INSTRUCTIONS

1. Half the cantaloupe and remove the seeds.

2. Use a small scoop or melon baller to scoop out the flesh of the cantaloupe into at least 12 melon balls.

3. Skewer two melon balls, two fresh basil leaves, and equally distribute the prosciutto and mozzarella among the six skewers.

4. Drizzle with the 2 Tbsp. of fresh pesto and enjoy right away.

NUTRITIONAL FACTS

- Calories: 162 kcal
- Fat: 11 g
- Carbohydrates: 5 g
- Protein: 11 g

2) Mini Bell Pepper Pizzas:

- Prep time: 10 minutes
- Cook time: 10 minutes
- Total time: 20 minutes
- Servings: 4
- Smart points: 2

INGREDIENTS

- 12 mini sweet peppers halved, seeded
- ½ cup pizza sauce
- ½ cup shredded mozzarella cheese
- ¼ cup mini pepperoni

INSTRUCTIONS

1. Preheat the oven to 400F. Place parchment paper on the baking sheet and set it aside.

2. Place small sweet peppers cut in half on a baking sheet. Fill with 1 tsp. pizza sauce, top with 1 tsp. cheese with a couple little slices of pepperoni.

3. Bake for 8-10 minutes, or until peppers soften and cheese melts.

NUTRITIONAL FACTS

- Calories: 18 kcal
- Carbohydrates: 1g
- Protein: 1g
- Fat: 1g

3) Air Fryer Coconut Shrimp with Sweet Chili Sauce:

- Prep time: 10 minutes
- Cook time: 25 minutes
- Total time: 35 minutes
- Serving: 1
- Smart points: 1

INGREDIENTS

- 2 large eggs
- 2 tablespoons lime juice
- 1 ½ cup coconut shavings, unsweetened or sweetened depending on preference
- ½ cup panko breadcrumbs
- ¼ cup all-purpose flour
- 1 teaspoon salt

- 1 teaspoon ground black pepper
- 1 teaspoon dried parsley
- Large 12-oz shrimp with the tail on, peeled

INSTRUCTIONS

1. If needed, preheat the air fryer to 375°F.
2. Whisk the eggs and lime juice in a medium-sized bowl and set it aside.
3. Mix the coconut, breadcrumbs, flour, salt, pepper, and parsley well in a separate medium-sized basin.
4. One at a time, dip each shrimp into the egg mixture, then drain and immediately dip it into the coconut mixture and press the coconut onto the shrimp if necessary.
5. Work in batches and arrange the shrimp in an air fryer basket in a single layer on a greased tray. Next, sprinkle the shrimp with nonstick or olive oil spray.
6. After 4 minutes of cooking at 375°F in the air fryer, turn the shrimp over and give them

another spray of nonstick or olive oil, then fry for a further 3 minutes, or until they are crispy and golden.

7. Depending on the quantity of shrimp you have and the size of your air fryer, remove the shrimp from the basket and repeat the cooking procedure if necessary.

8. Serve with your favorite sweet chili sauce and garnish with freshly chopped cilantro or parsley, if desired.

NUTRITIONAL FACTS

- Calories: 294 kcal
- Carbohydrates: 28g
- Protein: 21g
- Fat: 11g

4) Greek Yogurt Ranch Dip with Vegetables:

- Prep time: 3minutes
- Total time: 3 minutes
- Servings: 1
- Smart points: 1

INGREDIENTS

- 1 cup plain non-fat Greek yogurt
- 3/4 teaspoon garlic powder
- 1/2 teaspoon onion powder
- 1/2 teaspoon dried dill
- 1/4 teaspoon kosher salt
- 1/4 teaspoon Worcestershire sauce
- 1/8 teaspoon cayenne pepper
- Fresh chopped chives for garnish.

INSTRUCTIONS

1. Combine the Greek yogurt, garlic, onion, dill, salt, Worcestershire sauce, and cayenne in a medium-sized bowl.

2. Garnish with fresh chives and serve.

NUTRITIONAL FACTS

- Calories: 132 kcal
- Carbohydrates: 10g
- Protein: 21g
- Fat: 1g

5) Shrimp Scampi Stuffed Avocados:

- Prep time: 15 minutes
- Cook Time: 2 minutes
- Total Time: 17 minutes
- Servings: 1
- Smart points: 4

INGREDIENTS

- One pound of cooked tiny shrimp (40 to 50 counts); Tip: Purchase cleaned, cooked, and refrigerated shrimp from the butcher section of your grocery store to save time.
- 1 medium Roma tomato, diced very small
- 1/3 medium English cucumber, diced very small
- 1/3 cup red onion, diced very small
- 1/4 cup fresh cilantro, finely minced

- 2 to 3 tablespoons lime juice

- 1/2 teaspoon kosher salt, or to taste

- 1/2 teaspoon freshly ground black pepper, or to taste

- Hot sauce (I used two teaspoons of Cholula; you may also use Huichol) to taste

- 2 extra-large avocados or 3 average sized, halved and with about 50% of the flesh scooped out and put into the mixture

INSTRUCTIONS

1. Add all the ingredients to a large bowl, stirring to mix (if using raw shrimp, I suggest boiling cleaned shrimp for 1 minute or until just done, then chilling in an ice bath).

2. In terms of the avocados, you want to make the space between the avocado halves wider and somewhat hollowed out so that you can add the shrimp combination without making them completely clean.

3. Scoop out approximately 50% of the flesh and stir this into the shrimp mixture.

4. Taste the mixture and adjust with more salt, pepper, lime juice, hot sauce (I added two teaspoons, which gave it a bite, but not too spicy for us), and other seasonings to taste.

5. Once the avocados have been hollowed out, spoon the mixture inside and serve right away. Recipe is best fresh.

NUTRITIONAL FACTS

- Calories: 626 kcal
- Carbohydrates: 29g
- Protein: 57g
- Fat: 34g

6) Mini Wonton Appetizers with Various Fillings:

- Prep Time: 15 minutes
- Cook Time: 13 minutes
- Total Time: 28 minutes
- Servings: 24
- Smart points: 2

INGREDIENTS

- 1 lb Spicy Chorizo, bulk
- ½ teaspoon Kosher Salt
- 1 medium Sweet Onion, chopped
- 24 Wonton Wrappers
- 2 tablespoons Olive Oil, for brushing
- ¼- ⅓ cup Refried Beans
- 1 ½ cups Shredded Cheddar Cheese
- Sour Cream, optional

- Jalapeños, thinly sliced, optional

- Cherry Tomatoes, quartered, optional

- Additional Toppings - Guacamole and Salsa

INSTRUCTIONS

1. Preheat the Oven to 350°F. Add the spicy chorizo and sprinkle with salt to a large pan set over medium-high heat. Fry until browned. After removing from the pan, pat dry with paper towels.

2. Remove all except a few tablespoons of oil from the pan. When the onions are soft and transparent, add them to the skillet and cook for 4–5 minutes. After removing the pan from the heat, add the chorizo back along with the onions.

3. One at a time, brush both sides of the wontons, then carefully push each one into the little muffin tins.

4. Add 1 teaspoon of refried beans to the bottom of the wonton cup. Add a heaping tablespoon of the chorizo/onion mixture.

5. The muffin tin should be placed in an oven set to 350°F, cook the wontons for 10 to 13 minutes, or until the sides are well browned. Remove from the oven and add shredded cheese on top of each taco cup.

6. Taco cups should be taken out of the muffin tins and placed on a serving tray to prevent the bottoms from getting soggy.

7. Top with a dollop of sour cream, jalapeño slice and quartered cherry tomato (optional). Depending on your tastes, serve with more guacamole and salsa on the side..

NUTRITIONAL FACTS

- Calories: 241 kcal
- Carbohydrates: 16g
- Protein: 16g

- Fat: 12g

CHAPTER 7: SNACKS AND DESSERTS

1) Frozen Yogurt Bark with Berries and Granola:

- Prep time: 15 minutes
- Total time: 3 hours 15 minutes
- Servings: 12
- Smart points: 2

INGREDIENTS

- 2 cups whole milk vanilla yogurt
- ½ cup diced strawberries
- ¼ cup blueberries
- ¼ cup granola

INSTRUCTIONS

1. Apply wax or parchment paper to a rimmed baking quarter sheet.

2. After pouring the yogurt into the baking dish, distribute it uniformly to fit the shape of the baking sheet that has been ready.

3. Top with the strawberries, blueberries and granola.

4. Put the yogurt in the freezer for about three hours, or until it solidifies.

5. Cut into 12-15 pieces, and enjoy cold

6. Store leftovers in the freezer.

NUTRITIONAL FACTS

- Calories: 52 kcal

- Carbohydrates: 6g

- Protein: 2g

- Fat: 2g

2) Skinny Lemon Squares:

- Prep Time: 20 minutes
- Cook Time: 50 minutes
- Total Time: 1 hour 10 minutes
- Servings: 16
- Smart points: 3

INGREDIENTS

- 1 cup all-purpose flour, divided use
- ¼ cup cornmeal
- ⅛ teaspoon baking powder
- ⅛ teaspoon salt
- 2 large eggs
- 1 large egg white
- 1 teaspoon water
- 2 tablespoons butter, softened
- 1 cup granulated sugar, divided use
- 1 tablespoon lemon zest
- ½ cup lemon juice (about 4 lemons)

- 1 tablespoon confectioners' sugar

INSTRUCTIONS

1. In the middle of the oven, place an oven rack. Heat the oven to 350F degrees. Line an 8-inch square baking pan with foil, allowing the foil to extend over the rim by 2 inches. Spray the foil with non-stick spray.
    To make the crust:

2. In a small bowl, whisk together ⅔ cup of the flour, cornmeal, baking powder and salt until well blended; then set it aside.

3. In another small bowl, beat together the eggs and egg white.

4. Measure out 1 tablespoon of the egg mixture, put it in a cup, add the teaspoon of water, and mix. Set aside both egg mixtures.

5. With an electric mixer (affiliate link) on low speed, beat the butter in a medium bowl until creamy. Add a quarter of the cup of

granulated sugar and mix thoroughly. Beat in the egg-water mixture. Add the flour mixture and beat until blended. (The dough will be crumbly.)

6. Evenly press the dough mixture onto the bottom of the foil-lined pan and up the sides by ¼ inch. Bake until golden brown, 20 to 25 minutes.

Make the filling while the crust bakes:

7. Whisk together the remaining ⅓ cup flour and ¾ cup granulated sugar in a medium-sized bowl . Whisk in the remaining egg mixture until blended. Add the lemon zest and juice and blend well.

8. Take the crust out of the oven and set it aside on a rack. Reduce the oven temperature to 300F degrees. Over the hot crust, pour the lemon mixture. Bake for 20 to 25 minutes, or until the filling is set.

9. Take out of the oven and let cool on a wire rack. Refrigerate until cold, at least 1 hour and up to 8 hours.

10. When ready to serve, sprinkle the chilled bars with confectioners' sugar. Use the foil to lift the slab of bars from the pan. Cut into 16 even squares.

NUTRITIONAL FACTS

- Calories: 113 kcal
- Fat: 2g
- Carbohydrates: 22g
- Protein: 2g

3) Apple Crumble with Oat Topping :

- Prep time: 10 minutes
- Cook time: 45 minutes
- Total time: 55 minutes
- Servings: 10
- Smart points: 4

INGREDIENTS

- Apple Filling
- 2 lbs Apples (peeled, cored and diced in 1 inch cubes)
- 2 tablespoons Lemon Juice
- ¾ cup Granulated Sugar
- 1 teaspoon Ground Cinnamon
- ¼ teaspoon Ground Nutmeg
- ¼ teaspoon Ground Ginger
- ¼ cup All-purpose Flour
- Crumble Topping
- 1 cup All-purpose Flour

- 1 cup Oats (old-fashioned or instant
- 1 cup Brown Sugar
- 1 teaspoon Ground Cinnamon
- ½ teaspoon Ground Nutmeg
- ¾ teaspoon Baking Powder
- ½ teaspoon Salt
- ¾ cup Chilled Unsalted Butter (diced)

INSTRUCTIONS

Making apple filling :

1. Preheat the oven at 350°F (180°C).

2. Combine the diced and peeled apples with the granulated sugar, nutmeg, dried ginger, ground cinnamon, all-purpose flour and freshly squeezed lemon juice in a big bowl.

3. Give a gentle toss until the apples are coated well with sugar, flour and spices. Prepare the crumble topping and let the apple mixture rest for a bit .

Making Crumble Topping:

4. Combine the flour, oats, brown sugar, ground nutmeg, ground cinnamon, baking powder, and salt in a separate large bowl. All ingredients should be well mixed to create a crumb mixture.

5. Using your fingers, stir in the chilled unsalted butter cubes until the mixture comes together to form a crumbly topping.

Assembly and Baking :

6. Now, transfer the apple mixture to a greased cast iron skillet or a 10-inch round baking dish, spreading it out evenly (you may also use a 2-quart rectangle baking dish in place of the round one).

7. Evenly distribute the crumble topping over the apples.

8. Place it in the oven that has been preheated and bake for 40 to 45 minutes, or until the fruit is bubbling and the crumble has turned golden brown.

9. Before serving, let the crumble stand for a few minutes.

10. Serve warm or at room temperature with vanilla ice cream, whipped vanilla cream or custard

NUTRITIONAL FACTS

- Calories: 401 kcal
- Carbohydrates: 67g
- Protein: 3g
- Fat: 15g

4) Baked Apples with Cinnamon and Cranberries:

- Prep Time: 5minutes
- Cook Time: 40 minutes
- Total: 45 minutes
- Servings: 4
- Smart points:3

INGREDIENTS

- 1 cup chopped pecans
- ½ cup dried cranberries
- 4 tablespoons orange marmalade
- 2 tablespoon brown sugar
- 4 baking apples
- 4 tablespoons butter

INSTRUCTIONS

1. Preheat the oven to 350 degrees.

2. In a small bowl, combine the pecans, cranberries, orange marmalade, and brown sugar. Stir together until well mixed. Set aside.

3. Halve and remove the core from the apples. Transfer the halves ,cut side up, in a baking dish.

4. Place a pat of butter and some amount of the pecan-cranberry mixture inside each apple half.

5. Bake the apples for 30 to 40 minutes, or until they are soft. Regularly brush with collected pan juices.

6. Take out of the oven and let rest for approximately fifteen minutes.

7. Serve plain or with a scoop of vanilla ice cream.

NUTRITIONAL FACTS

- Calories: 502 kcal
- Carbohydrates: 61g
- Protein: 3g
- Fat: 31g

5) Dark Chocolate and Banana Pops:

- Prep time: 15 minutes
- Total time: 3 hours
- Servings: 6
- Smart points: 2

INGREDIENTS

- 3 large bananas, peeled
- 50g (1/2 bar) dark chocolate (70% – 90% cocoa)
- 2 Tbsp crushed salted pistachios (or any topping of your choice)

INSTRUCTIONS

1. Lay a piece of parchment paper on a small cookie sheet. Place chopped nuts or other toppings in a shallow dish and set aside.

2. Cut bananas in half across the width, then push a popsicle stick through the cut ends..

3. Break or chop chocolate into pieces and melt carefully over low heat (in a double boiler is best, but not necessary). Once melted, dip bananas into the chocolate, using a spoon to coat if needed.

4. Sprinkle your preferred toppings or nuts on the coated chocolate banana pop gently or add them to the chocolate.

5. Repeat with each banana, placing them on your parchment-lined sheet. You may drizzle any remaining chocolate on top! Place the tray in the freezer for 2-3 hrs.

6. Cool off with your frozen treat

NUTRITIONAL FACTS

- Calories: 150 kcal
- Carbohydrates: 20g
- Protein: 1g
- Fat: 5g

6) Spiced Pears with Greek Yogurt and Honey:

- Prep time: 10 minutes
- Cook time: 30 minutes
- Total time: 40 minutes
- servings: 2
- Smart points: 3

INGREDIENTS

- For the poached pears:
- 2 large Bosc pears
- 1 1-inch piece of freshly grated and peeled ginger
- 2 Tbsp honey
- 1.5 tsp ground cinnamon
  Adjust seasonings to taste:
- Plain Greek yogurt (benefits of Greek yogurt)
- Granola

- Chopped pistachios or other nuts and toppings

INSTRUCTIONS

1. Pears should be peeled, quartered, cored, and then added to water.

2. Simmer the liquid for 25 to 30 minutes, or until the pears are tender. You can determine if they're ready by poking them with a fork. There shouldn't be any resistance!

3. Take off from heat and let the pears cool in the liquid.

4. Top bowls of yogurt with 2 pear quarters. Granola, pistachios, a dash of cinnamon, some freshly grated ginger, and extra honey, if necessary, should be added. Feel free to use whatever toppings and seasonings you like!

NUTRITIONAL FACTS

- Calories: 250 kcal

- Carbohydrates: 40g

- Protein: 15g

- Fat: 5g

CHAPTER 8: DRINKS

1) Strawberry Mint Spritzer:

- Prep time: 5 minutes
- Total time: 5 minutes
- Servings: 1
- Smart points: 1

INGREDIENTS

- 4-5 fresh strawberries
- 1 cup sparkling water
- 1/2 lime, juiced
- 1 sprig fresh mint

INSTRUCTIONS

1. Muddle strawberries in a glass.
2. Add sparkling water, lime juice, and mint sprig.
3. Stir gently and serve over ice.

NUTRITIONAL FACTS

- Calories: 30 kcal
- Carbohydrates: 7g
- protein: 1g
- Fat: 0g

2) Citrus Cooler with Cucumber:

- Prep time: 5 minutes
- Total time: 5 minutes
- Servings: 1
- Smart points: 1

INGREDIENTS

- 1/2 grapefruit, juiced
- 1/2 orange, juiced
- 1 cup sparkling water
- 1 slice cucumber
- 1 sprig rosemary

INSTRUCTIONS

1. Combine grapefruit and orange juice in a glass.
2. Add sparkling water, cucumber slice, and rosemary sprig.
3. Stir gently and serve over ice.

NUTRITIONAL FACTS

- Calories: 80 kcal
- Carbohydrates: 20g
- Protein: 1g
- Fat: 0g

3) Spiced Iced Tea with Berries:

- Prep time: 10 minutes
- Cook time: 5 minutes
- Total time: 15 minutes
- Servings: 1
- Smart points: 1

INGREDIENTS

- 2 black tea bags
- 1 cup boiling water
- 1/2 teaspoon ground cinnamon
- 1/4 teaspoon ground cloves
- 1 cup ice
- 1/2 cup fresh berrie

INSTRUCTIONS

1. For five minutes, steep tea bags in hot water.

2. Remove tea bags and stir in cinnamon and cloves.

3. Let tea cool completely, then pour over ice in a glass.

4. Top with fresh berries.

NUTRITIONAL FACTS

- Calories: 70 kcal
- Carbohydrates: 15g
- Protein: 1g
- Fat: 0g

4) Green Tea Mango Smoothie:

- Prep time: 5 minutes
- Total time: 5 minutes
- Servings: 1
- Smart points: 3

INGREDIENTS

- 1 cup unsweetened green tea, chilled
- 1/2 frozen mango, chopped
- 1/2 cup Greek yogurt (2% fat)
- 1 tablespoon honey (optional)

INSTRUCTIONS

1. Blend all ingredients until smooth.
2. Add more ice if desired and serve immediately.

NUTRITIONAL FACTS

- Calories: 170 kcal
- Carbohydrates: 28g
- Protein: 15g
- Fat: 3g

5) Banana Chai Smoothie:

- Prep time: 5 minutes
- Total time: 5 minutes
- Servings: 1
- Smart points: 3

INGREDIENTS

- 1 frozen banana, sliced
- 1 cup unsweetened almond milk
- 1/4 cup chai tea concentrate
- 1 scoop protein powder (optional)
- 1/4 teaspoon ground cinnamon

INSTRUCTIONS

1. Blend all ingredients until smooth.
2. Add more ice if desired and serve immediately.

NUTRITIONAL FACTS

- Calories: 250 kcal
- Carbohydrates: 35g
- Protein: 20g
- Fat: 5g

CONCLUSION

Alright, my friend, we've reached the end of this tasty adventure with Nicole J. Deleon. Take a moment to savor the journey because, let's face it, life's too short for bland meals and boring diets.

In the grand finale, Nicole J. Deleon leaves you with this heartfelt nugget of wisdom: healthy eating is not about deprivation but a fiesta for your taste buds and your well-being. Every recipe here is like a flavor-packed high-five to your body and soul. Now, as you stride forward on your wellness path, remember, you're not just changing what's on your plate; you're weaving a narrative of self-care and delicious empowerment. Every meal is your canvas, and you're the artist of your health.

In the spirit of cheering you on, Nicole J. Deleon wants you to know that every little effort counts. Whether it's swapping out ingredients, trying a new recipe, or just relishing a mindful bite, each step is a victory. So, keep going, because you're rocking this wellness gig!

REVIEW

Hey there!

I hope this message finds you well. We'd love to hear your thoughts on The Ultimate Watch Your Weight Cookbook for Balanced Living 2024. Your feedback is invaluable to us and helps us continuously improve.

Could you spare a few moments to share your experience? Your insights mean the world to us, and we're eager to know how we can make things even better for you.

Your feedback is like a secret sauce that makes us better each day.

Thanks a lot!

Warm regards,

Nicole J. Deleon

www.ingramcontent.com/pod-product-compliance
Lightning Source LLC
Chambersburg PA
CBHW061639250726
48659CB00004B/1294